what is water?

what is water?

HOW YOUNG LEADERS CAN
THRIVE IN AN UNCERTAIN WORLD

Kayvan Kian

WHAT IS WATER?
How Young Leaders Can Thrive in an Uncertain World

ISBN   978-1-5445-0352-3   *Hardcover*
        978-1-5445-0350-9   *Paperback*
        978-1-5445-0351-6   *Ebook*

Cover design by Alex Robbins
Book design by John van der Woude
Graphic design by Robin van Merkestein and Tina Rataj
Author photograph by Giovanni Siani

"Per aspera ad astra"

—Latin phrase

*Dedicated to anyone who is
going through tough times.*

Table of Contents

Introduction

"*Learning how to think...really means learning how to exercise some control over how and what you think. It means being conscious and aware enough to choose what you pay attention to and to choose how you construct meaning from experience. Because if you cannot or will not exercise this kind of choice in adult life, you will be totally hosed.*"

—David Foster Wallace

Since the moment you were born, life has presented you with challenges and opportunities to work with. If all is going well for you, and you have full faith and trust you'll be able to deal with whatever comes along your path, then this book is not for you. You can set this book aside.

If, however, you do feel that your days can be too challenging for you at times, if you don't necessarily feel equipped to deal with everything that comes your way, or if you have any doubt that you can grow, thrive, and lead yourself and others through whatever is ahead as much as you would like to—then this book is for you.

This book contains exactly zero new ideas. Instead, you will find a synthesis of many ways of thinking that have helped people in real life grow stronger through their difficulties, whether two thousand years ago or just this morning. Throughout the chapters, you will find strong influences from Epictetus, Martin Seligman, Nassim Taleb, Marie Curie, Tim Ferriss, Julie and John Gottman, David Allen, Maryam Mirzakhani, Amelia Earhart, Seneca, Florence Nightingale, Bruce Lee, Ryan Holiday, Lao Tzu, and less well-known thinkers.

The goal is to offer something that is universal and simple—something of help to people of all ages—not with the intent of improving you or changing society but of giving you a sense that you have more choice, in any given moment, in any situation. You can therefore see this book as a good friend, a guide that helps you navigate and thrive wherever you are.

In the first chapter, you will find a perspective for how to view the world we all live in and the challenges it presents.

We then borrow a mindset from the ancient Stoics as a basis to deal with these challenges. After creating this common ground, the remainder of the chapters apply this basic mindset to a variety of themes, researched, brought together, and structured into the PERMA model by the thoughtful pioneer Martin Seligman.[1]

There is no one way to explore this book. You can read it from front to back, or only the chapters that appeal to you most. Feel free to pick and choose what is most relevant to you. Throughout the book, there are exercises allowing you to practice with the concepts we discuss. You can do these exercises in full, leave them for another time, or change them to your preference. It's your life, and this book is at your service.

The practical exercises you'll find have been tested over the course of seven years by thousands of participants in the Young Leaders Forum workshops around the world[2] and also by the author and other contributors. What you have in front of you is therefore the result of a collective collaboration, and it is exciting to share it all with you now as well.

Enjoy!

Awareness & Choice

～～～

ong ago, there lived a man named Daedalus, who was being held captive in a labyrinth on the island of Crete. Daedalus had built this labyrinth for Minos, the king of the island. Following a conflict with Minos, however, Daedalus had ended up imprisoned in his own creation. Being the brilliant craftsman and inventor that he was, Daedalus decided to build wings with which he would attempt to fly away and escape the island. He crafted one pair of wings from wax and feathers for himself, and another for his beloved son, Icarus. Before taking flight, Daedalus instructed his son to not fly too close to the sea, nor too high up toward the sun, but instead to follow Daedalus's lead in the middle. Once in the sky, however, the craftsman's words slowly slipped away from Icarus's mind as he got lost in the ecstasy of flying. As he drew closer to the sun, his wings began to melt. Once Icarus realized this, it was already too late. He plunged from great heights down into the sea.[1]

The story of Icarus is most commonly interpreted as a warning against hubris. Under this interpretation, the moral of the story is that if we overestimate ourselves and become arrogant like Icarus, we may very well create our own downfall.

However, consider this alternative interpretation: one could argue that there is nothing inherently wrong with "going higher"—or changing context—as long as one is equipped to match that context, which Icarus, with his wax wings, was not. How many of us feel like we are flying with wax wings, at times a little too close to the sun? How much of this situation is a consequence of your own choice, and how much of it seems to be a given?

What Is Water?

If we want to learn how to lead, grow, and thrive on a daily basis, where do we begin? A good place to start is context.

Each context that you're in requires a unique set of mind-sets, skills, and tools from you. You don't live in a vacuum or sterile laboratory—things happen continuously around you every day. As simple as this might sound, it is actually a very hard thing to become and remain aware of. The author David Foster Wallace illustrated this difficulty through a short story about an encounter between two young fish and an older fish. While swimming by, the older fish asks: "Morning, boys, how's the water?" Some time passes, after which one of the younger fish is puzzled and asks the other one: "What the hell is water?"[2]

In this chapter, we'll explore a way of becoming and staying more aware of our "water": the context we live in and its implications. This is an opportunity to lift yourself out of the water and have a fresh look at where you are. You can begin to see, examine, and name what constitutes the scenery of your life and start deciding on the changes that you want to make before plunging back in.

Let's start with a short exercise that aims to increase your awareness of your context.

A Closer Look at Water

Think about everything that has happened over the past six to twelve months and list the events that you still recall and that had an effect on you. The points you note can be positive or negative, local or global, etc. The following guiding questions may help.

Global Waters
- Which news headlines struck you in the last six to twelve months?
- What political and economic events are present in your mind?

Local Waters
- What happened in your region, city, and/or neighborhood?
- What have you grown accustomed to that was not part of your life a year ago?

Personal Waters
- What happened in your personal life and the lives of those around you?
- How is your life different today in comparison to a year ago?

Global Waters

Local Waters

Personal Waters

How the Water Feels

Take some time and reflect on the lists above. What feelings arise when you think about these events and situations? How do you think the people around you feel in the global and local waters that you described?

What's Happening?

Obviously, we don't have the chance to discuss your local or personal context, as they will be different for each person. However, we can work with the broadest common denominator that we have: the global context.

Our global waters can be described as VUCA: a world that feels, for many, to be volatile, uncertain, complex, and ambiguous.[3] The ultra-simplified way to describe this world would be:

- "Things are changing faster all the time."
  (Volatile, as opposed to stable.)
- "I have no clue what's happening next."
  (Uncertain, as opposed to certain.)
- "Everything is connected to everything else."
  (Complex, as opposed to simple.)
- "I don't even know what I need to know."
  (Ambiguous, as opposed to clear.)

You might say that things have always been this way. Even two millennia ago, Heraclitus said that "the only constant is change." However, one could argue that some periods in history have felt more VUCA than others. If you feel that the world around you is changing at a faster pace, and that you need to continuously expect the unexpected in a highly interconnected, unpredictable, and, at times, unclear world, then you most certainly are not alone.

Dreaming of Stability & Control

So what? Why does this matter? Well, one intuitively understands that such an environment can be a tremendous struggle for people. If we were to ask people whether they would like to have more volatility or less, many of them might say something along the lines of "I'm a pretty adventurous person, but it's okay for now, and less would be fine by me." Instead of volatility, they might prefer more stability, more certainty over uncertainty, simplicity over complexity, and clarity over ambiguity.

Aside from the obvious difficulties that a volatile, uncertain, complex, and ambiguous context presents, at the core of this struggle, there is an overwhelming sense of a lack of control. In general, people thrive in environments that they experience as stable and safe. The sense of being in control of our fate leads to better stress management, higher work performance, and even a stronger immune system. In contrast, a lack of this sense of control can lead to the opposite: higher rates of depression, stress and burnout, and lower rates of engagement.[4,5,6]

Thriving in a VUCA World

The purpose of this section is not to rub it in your face that it's all really difficult and then leave you on your own, wishing you the best of luck. Nor is the purpose solely to prevent you from collapsing under the pressures around you. This section is actually an invitation to turn it around and thereby put this predicament on its head: how can you lead, grow, and thrive in a VUCA world?[7]

To begin answering this question, where better to start than with people who, in your own view, have faced real challenges and are navigating the VUCA world with some success?

EXERCISE 2
Role Models Thriving in VUCA Waters

Think of someone whom you consider to be a role model, someone who has done or is doing something in the world that you admire. You are free to choose anyone: a neighbor, a sibling, a colleague, a friend, or someone you've read about in the news or seen on social media.

Once you've got someone in mind, take a few minutes to think about and make notes on these questions:

- What are some actions they take that you admire?

- What could their mindset be?

- How does this person help others navigate a VUCA world?

Analyzing one role model is a good start and can be insightful for you. However, what works for one person might not automatically work for someone else. What would happen if we were to analyze a large group of role models? What might they have in common?

What Happens in the Afternoon Will Happen in the Afternoon

If the common denominator for people who thrive in a VUCA environment is a unique mindset, then what could this mindset be? This is a mindset that was often taught amongst the ancient Stoics. In a nutshell, its essence can be formulated as "a radical focus on what you *can* control."

Indeed, let's repeat that one more time: a radical focus on what you *can* control.[8]

At any given moment in time, there are an infinite number of things outside of your control, while at the same time, there are also things that are within your control. How good are you at making a distinction between the two? We all have twenty-four hours in any given day. You can spend most of those hours—maybe justifiably so—being preoccupied with a wide array of things that are outside of your control. At the same time, you can invest an equal number of hours in the things that are actually within your control:

improving your own life and having a positive impact on your friends, family, colleagues, organization, neighborhood, society, etc.

This mindset has been passed on for generations. The ancient Stoics often recounted the tale of a person named Agrippinus. The story goes that one day, someone suddenly came to Agrippinus's house in the morning and told him that his fate would be determined by the Senate in a trial in the afternoon. In response to this news, Agrippinus went off for his daily exercise. When the people around him, surprised at his attitude, asked him how he could respond in such a way, of all the infinite responses available to him, Agrippinus said, "That's simple. I have built my life on one single motto: 'I do not add to my troubles.'" Agrippinus's trial was in the afternoon, and we can imagine that he might have thought something along the lines of "what happens in the afternoon will happen in the afternoon. But I refuse, with my own two hands and my own thoughts, to add anything on top of that, so who is up for some nice exercise?"[9]

Of course, it's not about the specific phrase. It's about the lens the phrase is hinting at; the mindset, so to speak. You could say, "I do not add to my troubles," or you can decide to have a radical focus on what you *can* control. Entrepreneurs often say, "I do what I can with what I've got," while others might live by "not in my control, not of concern." All of these phrases are hinting at the same mindset. You can use any one of these or create your very own—whatever helps you look at the world through this lens.

It is important to note, however, that this mindset is not an excuse for apathy. It is not about encouraging you to walk around without caring about what happens, shrugging off the ups and downs in your life. The aim of this lens is to empower you to achieve the opposite of apathy and help you cultivate an active attitude in life. This is about caring about your life so much that, by focusing on what you *can* control, you can invest all your thoughts, efforts, and energy in ways that work for you.

Now that we have discussed the central mindset, let's bring it further to life in the rest of the book through practical skills and perspectives that are *within* your control and positively contribute to leading, growing, and thriving in a VUCA world.

Chapter One—Essence

A fish can hardly see water. Our context is hard to notice precisely because it surrounds us everywhere, in every minute of every day.

The only constant is change. We live in times that, for many, feel very challenging due to their volatility, uncertainty, complexity, and ambiguity.

To thrive in a VUCA *world, maintain a radical focus on what you can control.* Be aware of where you are investing all your attention, heart, and energy.

> *"The sage is ready to use all situations and doesn't waste anything. This is called embodying the light."*
>
> —Lao Tzu

Positive & Negative

ne day, King Alexander the Great had a legendary encounter with Diogenes, a philosopher without any belongings. The king had heard many stories about Diogenes and wanted to meet him. After a long search, Alexander and his men found Diogenes sitting leisurely on the ground, leaning against a barrel. Alexander the Great approached him and said, "Diogenes, I have heard many great things about you. I would like to grant you any wish that you have." Hearing this, Diogenes looked up, thought for a moment, and answered, "Thank you. If I could make one wish, it would be for you to step to the left, so that you get out of my sun." Alexander the Great was struck and surprised by this simple response. His admiration for Diogenes only grew further, and he proclaimed to the crowd around him that "if I were not Alexander the Great, I would have wanted to be Diogenes."[1]

Sitting in Diogenes's Barrel

Why is this story still so appealing after thousands of years? Perhaps because Diogenes's reaction is so surprising. After all, what type of person would "fail" to take advantage of the opportunity to have any wish granted? This story can be interpreted in many ways. One interpretation is that Diogenes knew what he truly enjoyed and made sure that these things were also within his own sphere of control.

This chapter will attempt to do something similar, in order to increase the ratio of positive emotions in our lives.[2] Before we go further, it's important to be explicit about the following: this chapter is not intended to give the impression that negative emotions are "bad" and positive emotions are "good." There is a time and place for both. Negative emotions are an integral part of human life, and they have their own merits.[3] Instead, the question is whether, in the context of a VUCA world, you experience the ratio of positive emotions that you want to.

Let's take a closer look at the benefits of positive emotions. Experiencing positive emotional states can be considered a goal in itself—you really don't need to justify the fact that you want to feel good. However, positive emotions have a lot of great benefits, including:

- Broadening your focus and attention span
- Improving your problem-solving abilities
- Protecting your health and strengthening the immune system[4]

Moreover, experiencing positive emotions creates both a psychological and practical buffer that you might need on a rainy day. What does that mean? It is much easier to handle a negative event when you have a rich buffer of positive emotions which you have built over time, making you more resilient during tough times in life.

Many activities that create positive emotions (such as having fun with friends or being curious about a new topic) also have the positive side effect of building practical resources (social relationships, knowledge) that can help you during challenging times.[5] In sum, it's worth taking a closer look at positive emotions in your daily life and the lives of those around you.

Your Favorite Things

The good news is that it's possible to build your positive emotions buffer in an infinite number of ways. This book, of course, can't tell you what exactly it is that's going to give you a positive kick in life. That's for you to discover. What it can do is give you some directions on where to look.

Let's draw on some wisdom from the movie *The Sound of Music*. In this film, Julie Andrews plays the character of Maria, the governess of seven children. During a storm, she sits with them in their bedroom. The weather has scared the children, and, in order to soothe them, Maria starts singing about her favorite things:

Raindrops on roses
And whiskers on kittens
Bright copper kettles and warm woolen mittens
Brown paper packages tied up with strings
These are a few of my favorite things

Cream-colored ponies and crisp apple strudels
Doorbells and sleigh bells
And schnitzel with noodles
Wild geese that fly with the moon on their wings
These are a few of my favorite things

Girls in white dresses with blue satin sashes
Snowflakes that stay on my nose and eyelashes
Silver-white winters that melt into springs
These are a few of my favorite things

When the dog bites
When the bee stings
When I'm feeling sad
I simply remember my favorite things
And then I don't feel so bad[6]

This simple song conveys the wisdom of positive emotions and their helpful role in difficult times. You are now invited to create your own list of your favorite things.

EXERCISE 1
Small, Specific, Simple

Take a couple of minutes and create a list of your favorite things and activities. Try to be as specific as possible.

How did this exercise make you feel? What did you become aware of? What thoughts or ideas came up?

You might notice that, just like Julie Andrews, even thinking of your favorite things can invoke a positive feeling, which is what we would call savoring. By doing these types of exercises, and thereby becoming more aware of yourself, hopefully your palette of choice will also broaden. The more you are aware of your favorite things, the better you can integrate them into your day-to-day experience and not leave them up to chance. However, which of your favorite things are actually *within your control*?

EXERCISE 2

Small, Specific, and Simple, with a Radical Focus on What You Can Control

Take another look at your list, this time looking at it from the perspective of "a radical focus on what you can control." Which of the items could you experience in the coming two to three weeks, if you wanted to? Draw a star next to these actionable favorite things.

If you have at least one star, that's great news. In the context of a VUCA world, positive emotions matter, and there is at least one favorite thing that is within your control. For now, that's enough.

If you decide that you'd like to work on it, here are a number of things you could do in order to make it a bit easier or more likely for you to pursue these favorite things:

- Keep adding items to your favorite things list.
- Create time and space in your day for your favorite things.
- Find ways to remind yourself of your favorite things in your daily life.

Alright. So far, so good. But what if we press pause for a moment and put on our cynical hat?

- A walk on the beach
- A nice cup of coffee in the sun
- A chat with your kids
- A moment of spontaneous beauty
- A boost of extra sleep
- A funny video

We could very well say: "Well...this is nice and all, but it's also quite trivial. I'm not going to spend much thought on this, let alone devote entire sections of my time to this. I actually have a job to do. I have lists of things to take care of and to worry about."

Well, that sounds pretty convincing, but is it really true?

On a more philosophical level, what this exercise is asking is: You are a human being, living and walking on this earth, so what makes you happy? How well do you know that about yourself? And how easy or difficult are you making it for yourself to actually experience those things? And how okay are you with that answer?

Also, what does all of this mean for how you interact with others (who are navigating the same VUCA context)? How well do you know what other people's favorite things are? How well could you write that list of favorite things for your family members? What about the five people with whom you work the most? What's the least you can do to help them with their favorite things?

Of course, you could argue that the people around you are responsible for their own happiness. You don't necessarily need to take responsibility for other people's favorite things to happen. However, the least you could do is a "step zero" type of approach: that is, to at least not get in their way (too often) by assuming that your favorite things are universal.

"Step zero" questions:

- Is your favorite topic of conversation also theirs?
- Is your idea of a wonderful afternoon or a celebration also theirs?
- What would they love to do if they had a day off?
- What are they most looking forward to right now?

The Positive of the Negative

So far, we've looked at using simple awareness of our favorite things, followed by intentional action, as one way of experiencing more positive emotions in our lives.

This chapter, however, is not about pretending to be happy when you feel down. Some might say that negative emotions are intrinsically bad, because they often arise from negative situations and they feel unpleasant. As understandable as that argument might sound, it's good to consider what the value and benefits of negative emotions could be.

EXERCISE 3

The Merits of Negative Emotions

Can you recall an instance where you experienced a negative emotion that had merit for you or helped you realize or do

---

something you wouldn't have realized or done otherwise? Think about this instance and explore the following questions:

- What negative emotion(s) did you feel in that situation?

- What effect did they have on you?

- How did they help you overcome the situation at hand?

Negative emotions are an integral part of human nature; cutting them out altogether would remove an enormous and rich part of our experience. Emotions help us clarify our goals and values—we learn what's important to us by observing how we react to what happens in our lives.

All emotional states—the negative as well as the positive—can open certain avenues and possibilities, while closing others. In this case, negative emotions can be a strong motivator. We often act most decisively and persistently to remove the causes of negative emotions. Also, somewhat surprisingly, taking some "time out" when you feel bad can also be beneficial for you. By taking time to rest, you are allowing your body to rebuild strength.[7]

That being said, in a VUCA world, it's not always apparent how negative something really is. If you don't take the time to assess upsets, it's easy to get overwhelmed with the amount of exposure to negativity that you might have through work, social media, email, news, and voice and text messages.

Is Everything Forever Personal?

Therefore, in the following section, like seasoned mathematicians, we will focus on ways to increase the ratio of positive emotions simply by decreasing the level of what can be called "unnecessary negativity" in our lives—in other words, "clearing out the noise."

Decrease Your Exposure (Quantity)

A quite straightforward way of going about this is to limit your exposure to things that give rise to negative experiences or feelings—in other words, to create your "optimal level of distance" to sources of negativity.[8]

EXERCISE 4

What's That Sound?

Write down a list of things in your daily life that give rise to negative emotions in you. Think of places, media, people, and thoughts that are not worth the extra negativity that they bring into your life. Next, put a star next to the ones you could afford to limit or stop completely.

Decrease the Impact
of the Exposure (Quality)

After you've decreased your exposure to sources of negativity that you'd like to do without, the question that remains is: how could you limit the negative impact of all the shocks and "stings" that are still left?

The concept that will be introduced here is that of learned optimism.[9] This concept is about how you evaluate and interpret events that happen in your day-to-day life. It is not about making things seem better than they are; rather, it is about not making them seem worse (in the spirit of Agrippinus's motto, "I do not add to my troubles"). Let's practice this concept through an example.

EXERCISE 5
The Wedding Speech

Imagine you have been asked to give a surprise wedding speech together with your cousin. It's not just any wedding, but the wedding of your niece. One night, late after work, you finally finish writing the speech. You have spent a lot of time on it and worked many days to make it perfect. Reading through the whole speech again, you feel proud of what you have created. You send it to your uncle, who you hope will be proud of and impressed by your work.

The next morning, on your way to work, you see that you have received a voice message from your uncle. You listen to the voice message with excitement, waiting for your uncle's praise and enthusiasm. Instead, you hear the following message:

"Hi. I received the speech. I didn't like it. Please call me back."

Take a moment and note down what thoughts and emotions come to your mind.

Whenever something happens in our life, whether we want it or not, we will experience it on at least three dimensions. This happens automatically—often, we are not even aware of it—and will trigger an emotional reaction. These three dimensions are:

- *Subject*: Personal versus impersonal
- *Scope*: Everything versus specific
- *Time*: Forever versus temporary[10]

Let's look at these dimensions by interpreting the wedding speech example across each of them.

1. Personal versus Impersonal

One way to interpret the wedding speech message is to take it completely personally, as if there is something wrong with us, a human flaw or deficit that needs to be fixed. In the voice message, while we may hear "I did not like it," what we are thinking is "We all know what he means. Who does he not like? It's obviously me! He's probably thinking 'I don't know who asked you to give this speech. It's really bad. I can't believe that you aren't able to do such a simple thing.'"

On the other hand, if we interpret the message on the far-right end of the continuum in a completely impersonal way, then we interpret it as: "He did not like the speech, and that's all." Perhaps he had given some ideas for the content or style of the speech that you hadn't incorporated in the way he envisioned it, and he wants to add those elements.

2. Everything versus Specific

What does your uncle mean by "it," anyway? The entire speech? Really? He didn't like the structure, the jokes, the anecdotes, the tone, the length, and everything else?

Or, maybe, there was just one joke that he found inappropriate.

3. Forever versus Temporary

Finally, the effect of your terrible speech may have permanently affected your relationship with your uncle. He may see you in a different light forever—as an idiot. In fact, your uncle might have already talked with other family members about your speech in the meantime. It's probably a huge disappointment in their eyes. In the future, nobody from the family will dare to ask you to give a speech anymore, and slowly, you might end up being irrelevant to the family—the only group you truly feel like you belonged to.

Or, just maybe, your uncle will be happy when you call back. This isn't the first family incident, and of course, "this too shall pass."

This exercise is, once again, not about making things seem better than they are. It can be very unhelpful to make whatever happens seem impersonal, specific, and temporary when it's not. It's therefore not about putting a smile on your face, when all the while you actually feel like hiding under a blanket and crying. Instead, it is about helping you not interpret things as worse than they actually are and, hence, clearing out all the noise. In other words, this exercise is about realizing that you have a choice.

Many situations can be highly ambiguous, and much communication is often incomplete. To be clear, your initial interpretation across the three dimensions could exactly correspond with the reality of the situation. Also, there might be benefits to overestimating negative signals, just to be on the safe side. However, if you interpret each signal in a VUCA world in a highly "personal," "everything," and "forever" way, it can become overwhelming and too much to bear.

So, what are your options?

Option #1

Immediately after hearing your uncle's message, you could call your cousin in a state of panic. You tell him, "Our uncle didn't like the speech."

If you do that, what do you think will happen next? Probably the same thing that happened to you. Your cousin will interpret the situation on the same three dimensions. Consequently, your cousin might call your uncle in a state of anger and start the conversation in an unnecessarily harsh and negative tone. Research shows that this is one of the strongest indicators that a conversation will also finish on a harsh and negative tone.[11]

Events like these are comparable to an oil spill—an energetic oil spill, if you will. This type of energy can move at a high speed through groups of people, whether it's a family, an organization, a neighborhood, or a group of friends.

So, what now? Let's rewind this scenario and realize that we have a choice.

Option #2

Before talking to your cousin, you could, for instance, take a breath and try to understand what might be really bothering you. Do a quick check on each of the three dimensions. Challenge yourself by asking how far off your immediate reaction might be from reality. Call your uncle to check with him how bad things actually are and discuss possible solutions, thereby preventing the oil spill in your family interaction.

EXERCISE 6
Reality Check

Think about a recent upsetting incident from the past month. What happened?

Now, reflect on your initial response and position it along each of the three dimensions:

Personal   **Impersonal**

⟵——————————————————————⟶

- Was it about you?
- Was it only about you?
- Was it about something else? If so, what?

Everything   **Specific**

⟵——————————————————————⟶

- Did it concern an isolated issue or did it affect other areas as well?
- Did you need to change everything or only parts of it?
- What was the core issue and its implications?

Forever   **Temporary**

$\longleftrightarrow$

- Did this incident have any mid- to long-term consequences?
- How many people are still raising the incident?
- Did the incident have any positive side effects or "collateral beauties?"[12]

Now, looking back with everything you know, note where you think "reality" was in that moment. How close or far was this from your first response?

The Best of Both Worlds

Each of us has our own tendencies to interpret events on a certain end of a spectrum. Some of us might frequently take things personally; others often engage in what can be called "forever thinking," and still others don't pause to specify the exact problem. Not all of these tendencies are necessarily within our immediate control. Some of them could be part of upbringing, personal experiences, or the belief that—at times—it can be better to be safe than sorry. The main question here is: how much reflection time do you allow yourself between events and your conclusions about them?

By the way, this applies equally to positive incidents (such as a compliment, something going your way, or a major success).

How easy or difficult are you making it for yourself to experience an event's true positivity on the three dimensions?

- *Impersonal:* "Anybody could have done it."
- *Specific:* "I only worked on a small part of it."
- *Temporary:* "People will forget anyway."

If you interpret every negative event too far on the left side of these three scales, and every positive one too far on the right, it's a bit of the worst of both worlds.

Knowing that the same applies to others, you could take this into consideration when communicating. How clearly are you positioning reality for others on the three dimensions? How much are you leaving others guessing?

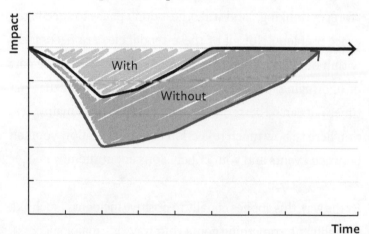

Dip Less Deep & Recover Faster

As you can imagine, mastering this can require some effort. At the same time, adopting techniques that *are* within your control can help you be affected less deeply and recover more quickly from a continuous stream of random negative events in a VUCA world.

When All Else Fails

So far, we've become more aware of how to build up a buffer with our favorite things, and how to make the dips from negativity less deep and the recovery faster.

Now, imagine a scenario in which you've run out of your buffer. Perhaps there hasn't been much opportunity, time, or energy to do any of your favorite things. It also doesn't seem like that's going to change anytime soon. You might even have negative reserves at the moment. And actually, you can't reduce the negativity of your situation any more. You've taken out the unnecessary noise, and it's still pretty bad.

In such moments, is there still a positive emotion that you can tap into, independent of where you are, what's going on, how bad things are, whom you're with, and all other variables?

If the answer were yes, how helpful would that be?

In order to figure this out, let's zoom out for a moment and look at broad types of positive emotions. Here's one possible overview of positive emotions (feel free to add to this list):

Affection	Curiosity	Hope	Passion
Awe	Delight	Inspiration	Relief
Comfort	Enthusiasm	Joy	Satisfaction
Compassion	Freedom	Love	Serenity
Confidence	Gratitude	Optimism	Wonder

EXERCISE 7
Tapping into New Sources

Take a moment to think about which role these types of emotions play in your life. How often do you experience them? Are there any emotions you would like to experience more often?

Realizing that there are different types of positive emotions might help broaden your choice of which ones you want to tap into. You might realize, looking back at that list of your favorite things, that they mainly give you certain types of positive emotions while skipping others.

However, so far, we haven't answered our opening question yet. Which positive emotion is most within our control, when all else fails? While the answer may vary from person to person, the emotion that many thinkers feel is most in our control is gratitude. Even in the most difficult of circumstances, human beings have been capable of experiencing gratitude in their own unique and private way.[13] Perhaps it's not a surprise that through the centuries and across cultural and geographic boundaries, many of our great traditions are about the cultivation of gratitude.

We could talk about gratitude for a long time, but the best way to understand the accessibility and the effect of gratitude is by experiencing it. So, let's move on to our next exercise.

EXERCISE 8
Gratitude Letter

Think about someone who has had a significant positive impact on your life. This could be someone who is still with you

---

or not, an old schoolteacher, someone from your office or your personal life; it could be someone you have spoken with or never met in real life. The point is to choose someone.

You are now invited to write this person a letter (you don't need to share it with them), describing what you are grateful for, specifically, and why. If you don't know how to begin, just start with the first sentence that comes to mind.

GRATITUDE LETTER

How did it feel to do this? What did you notice while writing?

Hopefully, this exercise has helped you realize that you can tap into an infinite source of gratitude all by yourself. It might also have given you insight into your most important needs.

You, as a human being, are able to access a sense of gratitude for things that don't necessarily have anything to do with your here and now. In other words, you can tap into a source of positive emotions that does not require your current circumstances to always be pleasant, comfortable, or stress-free. This invitation is not necessarily for moral reasons, such as "you must be grateful" or "you must feel X amount of gratitude in order to be a good person," but for pragmatic ones. All you need is a radical focus on what you are grateful for.

Deliberate Deprivation

If gratitude is so great, why aren't we all experiencing it all the time? The ancient Romans and Greeks were well aware of the following truth: as humans, we are incredibly good at getting used to what we have. Think of how good you feel the first day you achieve or obtain something that you have wanted for a long time. How does the first day of achieving or having this differ from the sixteenth week? We often adjust to what we have quite easily.

In one way or another, many ancient cultures and traditions promoted a practice that could be called *deliberate deprivation*.[14] Consciously removing the presence of something you might take for granted, for a limited (previously decided upon) period of time, is a way of ensuring that you won't take it for granted anymore.

For example, if you take heating for granted when it's cold, how about shutting off the heat for a week? If you take your shoes for granted, how about leaving home without them for a day? If you take your means of transportation for granted, how about living without it for a month?

Short-term, deliberate deprivation works like a reset of sorts. Instead of getting stuck in a treadmill where the things you have don't seem to be enough, you could opt for a lifestyle of "resetting." This way you become better aware of what you have and how much "you would wish that you had what you have, if you didn't have it anymore."

If for any reason you would prefer not to remove anything in the external world, it can often be enough to visualize being without that which is dear to you—a thought experiment that is also *always within your control*.

Unpacking the Present

In the previous exercise, we practiced experiencing gratitude for the past. Let's now apply the same skill to the present.

Every moment that you experience has a potentially infinite number of factors that make its existence possible in the first place. Learning to unpack the present means becoming more aware of those factors, and how something specific can be seen as an inseparable part of the whole. For example, as you are reading this sentence, think of three things that make it possible for you to do so. Now, think of three more that are less obvious.

You can apply this exact same technique to something you're grateful for in the present in the following exercise.

EXERCISE 9
Unpacking Gratitude

Take a moment to think about these questions...

- What do you deeply value about the here and now?

- What would you miss if you didn't have it anymore?

- What do you appreciate not having in your surroundings?

- What are all the things that support your answers to these questions?

Whether the things you are grateful for belong to the past or to the present, the good news is that your experience of gratitude always takes place in the *here and now*. And by the way, have you ever been anywhere else, other than the here and now?

Chapter Two—Essence

Enjoy your favorite things. Like a buffer, the positive emotions we experience can help us deal better with daily negative events. And they feel good.

Clear out the noise. You can reduce "unnecessary negativity" by decreasing your exposure, and by performing reality checks: personal versus impersonal, everything versus specific, and permanent versus temporary.

Unpack your presents. Gratitude is a positive emotion that is always there for you to access. Whether you focus on the past or the present, there is an infinite list of things to choose from.

"The thankful receiver bears a plentiful harvest."
—William Blake

Strengths & Weaknesses

"What kind of a man do you suppose Heracles would have become if it hadn't been for the famous lion, and the hydra, the stag, the boar, and the wicked and brutal men whom he drove away and cleared from the earth? What would he have turned his hand to if nothing like that had existed? Isn't it plain that he would have wrapped himself up in a blanket and gone to sleep? First of all, then, he would surely never have become a Heracles if he had slumbered the whole of his life away in such luxury and tranquility; and even if he had, what good would that have been to him? What would have been the use of his

arms and all his strength, endurance, and nobility
of mind if such circumstances and opportunities
hadn't been there to rouse him and exercise him?"[1]

—Epictetus

Riding the Waves of Flow

There are moments in life where we become so absorbed in the task at hand that we enter a unique state. This experience is not necessarily positive or negative. It is a state that Mihaly Csikszentmihalyi once famously defined as "flow," and it's what we'll explore in this chapter.[2,3]

In a state of flow, you aren't concerned with the past or future. Instead, your consciousness merges with the activity to such an extent that even your experience of time is altered. Some people experience flow while playing the guitar, while others do while solving math problems, running, painting, reading a book, or cooking.

Being in a state of flow comes with many benefits, including increased performance and creativity, higher self-esteem, more emotional stability, higher energy levels, and lower stress levels. People often feel an intense sense of accomplishment when they look back at what they've accomplished while "in flow." Furthermore, it's much harder for negative emotions to find their way in when your mind is purely focused on the task at hand, without thought of the past or the future.[4]

"Okay," you're probably thinking. "I've got it. But how do I get into that state?" In the same spirit as Heracles, one very practical way of entering flow is by matching your strengths with the challenge at hand.[5] This sounds very simple, but there are numerous barriers that can get in the way of actually doing it, including a lack of:

- Awareness of what you're good at and what energizes you
- A shared language by which you can describe the specific activities you are good at and that give you energy
- Practical opportunities to do those things

The next section will provide the tools for overcoming these barriers.

A Framework for Strengths[6]

Let's start by figuring out what strengths actually are, by drawing two simple lines: one horizontal, one vertical.

Truism #1

There are certain things in life you're not so good at, and there are certain things you're better at.

Very bad ←———————————————→ Very good

Truism #2

At the same time, there are also certain things in life that drain your energy, and there are certain things that energize you.

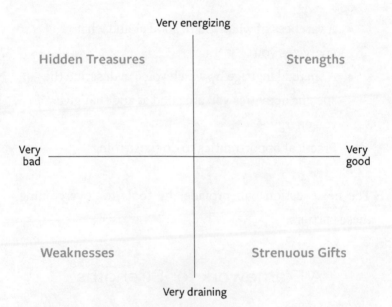

With these four boxes, we now have a simple structure to explore. Let's have a closer look at each part.

Strengths

There are things that you are good at and which give you energy. This is what you could call "strengths." Depending on the person, this can be any skill: creativity, listening, solving problems, humor, detail orientation, etc. When you apply your strengths on a level not so challenging that it burns you out and not so simple that it bores you (remember Heracles), that's where the magic happens. This is where you can reap the benefits of being "in the flow."

This chapter is an invitation to find more hours in a week to apply your strengths in different settings of your life. Of course, there can be a point at which you begin overusing them or applying them in misplaced contexts. Chances are, however, that at this moment, you are underusing them.

EXERCISE 1

Discovering Strengths

Take a moment to list as many of your strengths as you can. For instance, when did you work hard for a great result and feel like you could continue forever? What skills were you using in that moment?

Strenuous Gifts

"Strenuous gifts" are a particularly paradoxical combination: things that you are good at, but that at the same time drain your energy. Again, this can be any skill, depending on the person. There is a risk of mistaking this category for a strength, if you only take into consideration what you're good at. It is easy to imagine that you might end up using them a lot precisely because you are good at them, without acknowledging how depleted you might feel after using them. Something that drains you is, by this definition, definitely not a strength.

Spend your time in this category with moderation. You're good at performing your strenuous gifts; they benefit you and the people around you. They probably help you accomplish a lot of tasks. But keep your energy in mind. Using your strenuous gifts too much can be a recipe for burnout. You can only imagine how someone who spends the better part of their (work)days in that quadrant must feel in the evenings.

EXERCISE 2

Noticing Strenuous Gifts

Take a moment to list as many of your strenuous gifts as you can. For instance, when did you receive praise for something you did well yet really disliked doing? What skills were you using in these moments?

Hidden Treasures

There are also things that you're not so good at, but, interestingly enough, they do energize you. This is what you could call "hidden treasures." Why? Spending time in this quadrant can be fun, enjoyable, relaxing, and even exciting—all of which can give you the needed energy to better deal with challenging times. Moreover, the fact that you enjoy it could also be a hint of a talent, i.e., a dormant strength.

The least you can do with this category is acknowledge it and enjoy your time in it. Find environments where you can explore your hidden treasures. This category could also be an invitation for you to develop new strengths. If you've hit the ceiling of getting better at your strengths, this could be a good garden to grow your future ones with the proper practice, attention, and opportunity.

EXERCISE 3
Finding Hidden Treasures

Take a moment to list as many of your hidden treasures as you can. For instance, what are things you enjoy doing even if you are not currently good at them? What skills are you using in these moments?

Weaknesses

Weaknesses are the intersection of what could be seen as a clear mismatch: those things that you're not good at and (if that's not bad enough) also drain your energy. There are different ways of dealing with weaknesses. You can decide to improve all or some of them, ignore them, embrace them, avoid them, or get rid of them altogether (in a magical world). However, as we've discussed earlier, our main goal here is to find ways to thrive in an already challenging world. Given that the use of weaknesses can be a barrier to getting into flow, you could therefore think about ways to minimize the hours spent using them.

But what if, for some reason, you actually do need to perform based on your weaknesses? In that case, you could ask yourself: what is the minimum skill level (varying from zero to Olympic level) you need to elevate your weaknesses to, so that they don't stand in the way of you reaching your goals? If, for instance, you have to briefly speak in public, and you're neither good at it nor enjoy it, what would be the bare minimum you need to learn? Try to define what you need to learn for those five-minute presentations, not what you need in order to become a talk show host.

A highly efficient way of minimizing weaknesses is compensating for them with strengths to achieve your goals: *minimizing by maximizing*. If, for example, you want to entertain, teach, or inspire large groups of people and public speaking is a weakness, perhaps you can accomplish the same goal by focusing on writing (if that is a strength). Or, if you find it difficult to organize a fun day with your family because you're not very creative, you might be able to notice and pick up on ideas over time using your listening skills (if that is a strength) in order to accomplish that same goal.

EXERCISE 4
Listing Weaknesses

Take a moment to list as many of your weaknesses as you can. For instance, what activities have you not been good at and have you never enjoyed for as long as you can remember? What skills were you trying to use in those moments?

EXERCISE 5

Putting It All Together

For a more thorough assessment of your strengths (S), strenuous gifts (SG), hidden treasures (HT), and weaknesses (W), you can fill out the following chart.[7] Feel free to add any additional skills you have to the list. You can even plot them in a matrix (by drawing your own or using Appendix A).

Skill	Good at? (y/n)	Energizing? (y/n)	S	SG	HT	W
Adapting: Being flexible to the demands of a changing situation						
Advocating: Supporting and arguing for a cause						
Ambition: Setting and working toward high goals						
Authenticity: Being yourself, independent of the price you pay for it						
Building Relationships: Investing in strong and long-term bonds						
Caring: Helping and taking care of others						
Coaching: Guiding others to solve personal or professional challenges						
Competing: Comparing yourself with and outperforming others						
Conceptual: Identifying abstract patterns and relevant information in complex and unstructured situations						

Skill	Good at? (y/n)	Energizing? (y/n)	S	SG	HT	W
Courage: Overcoming your fears with emotional strength to pursue your goals						
Creativity: Coming up with new and ingenious approaches to complete a task or solve a problem						
Detail Orientation: Zooming in on the details of things and activities						
Discipline: Accurately following procedures and rules						
Emotional Awareness: Being aware of your own and others' emotional states						
Entrepreneurship: Identifying opportunities and acting upon them						
Focusing: Dedicating attention and energy to a single task at a time						
Humor: Focusing on the amusing and comical aspects of what is						
Interest: Exploring, learning, and discovering new themes in life						
Listening: Attending to what others have to say and share						
Motivating: Getting others to take action toward reaching goals						
Networking: Establishing connections with and between people						
Organizing: Structuring the planning and execution of tasks						
Personal Development: Developing and improving yourself						
Planning: Thinking through practical steps to reach a goal						

Skill	Good at? (y/n)	Energizing? (y/n)	S	SG	HT	W	
Pragmatism: Dealing with problems in a practical, action-oriented way							
Public Speaking: Speaking in front of and conveying your message to an audience							
Resilience: Recovering from difficulties and persisting through challenging conditions							
Resourcefulness: Mobilizing resources in an unconventional and creative way							
Risk Management: Foreseeing risks and deciding how to deal with them							
Solving Problems: Identifying issues and finding solutions							
Strategy: Selecting the best possible approach to increase the odds of success							
Teaching: Translating knowledge, ideas, and situations in ways that others can understand							
Teamwork: Working with groups of people							
Visionary: Imagining an ideal future							
Writing: Putting your ideas and messages on paper							

By going through the list step by step, you might discover that things you thought were your strengths or weaknesses might fall into other categories. If you want to, you could also get together with people who know you well and ask them about their perspectives.

Just as one can have an X-ray of their physical body, this exercise tries to help you take an X-ray of your skillset. Can this "X-ray" change over time? Most likely it will. With practice, hidden treasures can turn into strengths. If you overuse a strength to the point that it wears you out, it could become a strenuous gift. In a different context, a weakness could actually become fun and turn into a hidden treasure. However, as much as things can change over time, the important question right now is how to do more of the things you're good at and that give you energy today.

EXERCISE 6

Using Your Compass

You now have a compass to manage your energy better throughout the day and match your strengths better with the tasks at hand. With this compass, you can therefore increase the chances of entering the state of flow. Reflect on the following questions, noting down anything that comes to mind.

- How can you use your strengths more often?

- How can you moderate the use of your strenuous gifts?

- How can you enjoy and develop your hidden treasures?

- How can you minimize the use of your weaknesses?

When One Size Doesn't Fit All

According to ancient Greek mythology, there once lived a very "hospitable" man called Procrustes. Every traveler passing by his house was invited into his home to stay over for the night.

There was only one catch to this. The travelers had to fit *exactly* in the bed they would sleep in—not metaphorically, but literally. Meaning that if they were too short, he would stretch them out. If they were too tall, he would cut off a part of them. By whatever means necessary, all the people passing by the "hospitable" Procrustes's house would end up being the exact same size—however, in a somewhat deformed way.[8]

How much do you expect others to have the same strengths and weaknesses as you do? How well could you fill out the strengths assessment for the friends and colleagues you interact with most? When you're requesting something from someone, how much do you play into their strengths? When you are giving people advice, are you only trying to improve their weaknesses?

The same lens can be applied to groups of people. Do you, as a team or family, have a unique set of strengths or weaknesses? What are the advantages or risks that you have as a group? How could this affect the way you work and live together? Can you imagine ways of getting more in the flow as a group, while at the same time accomplishing what is important to you?

Chapter Three—Essence

Get into the flow. You can become so absorbed in the activity of the moment that time stands still. Not only is flow a unique experience in itself, it also has numerous benefits that help you thrive in a VUCA world.

Enter with strengths. There are many doorways into flow. One that is within your control is using your strengths on a level not so challenging that it burns you out, but also not so easy that it bores you.

Increase the chances. You can aim to increase the hours per week in which you use your strengths by moderating your strenuous gifts, enjoying and developing your hidden treasures, and minimizing your weaknesses.

"Be like water."

—Bruce Lee

You & Others

~~~

thena was the ancient Greek goddess of wisdom. She was the guardian of many cities and the helper of heroes. When one of these heroes, Odysseus, king of Ithaca, was traveling back home under challenging circumstances, she would often watch over him. In a famous instance, when Odysseus needed to travel without being noticed, Athena helped him disguise himself, changing his clothes and even his appearance. In other instances, Athena would put strength and courage into his heart, empowering him just enough for him to continue his journey.[1,2]

Taking Everything Away
That Isn't the Statue

As history has shown, social life is an integral part of human life. The term "social life" is quite broad and could refer to a great many things. In this chapter, we'll zoom in using a narrower definition.

Someone once asked the great artist Michelangelo, "How do you create your statues?" His response was quite surprising: "Well, that's quite easy. First, I take a piece of marble. Then, I take away everything that isn't part of the statue I'm trying to create. What remains is the statue."[3]

If the broad term "social life" is a large piece of marble, let's start by clarifying what this chapter doesn't consider to be part of the statue for now:

- Having over five thousand people in your address book
- Frequent invitations to interesting events
- A sense that you are "popular" and that people like you instantly

Some of these qualities and descriptions might sound familiar to you, and they can be very beneficial. However, if we take away many of the different forms that human interactions can take on in daily life, what remains is the one thing we want to focus on in this chapter, namely the sense that there is someone in the world who cares about you.[4]

People who experience that there's someone in the world who cares about them can cope significantly better with life challenges than those who don't. Most of us sense intuitively that having somebody who cares about us is an essential component of life. Especially in a VUCA world, the sense of *not* being alone serves as a buffer for many challenges. It can help you cope with disappointments, keep your mind sharp, help you through tough times, and even boost your physical health.[5]

If you are one of those people who has two, three, or even five of those individuals in your life, even better. These people can be anyone—a family member, a partner, a friend, even a colleague to whom you've grown close. What can this look like? It can take on myriad forms. Some examples are:

- You can call this person for support when you're having a bad day.
- This person often makes decisions with your interest in mind.
- These people help you out in crucial moments of your career.
- This friend is here for you whenever you need him/her, even at 3:00 a.m.

The central feature here is that you *feel* cared for. The source or potential sources of caring can be wide-ranging. This chapter won't be defining this for you, but rather will help you create awareness of what these things could be.

If you have been paying attention, you may notice what appears to be a problem. The central philosophy of this book is "a radical focus on what you *can* control." How much is it in your control for others to care about you? How successful would you be if you were to ask somebody on the street to care about you from that moment onwards?

Let's assume that this is not possible at all. How should we address this difficulty? Do we say, "Not in my control, not of concern," so we might as well skip this chapter altogether? Or is there an elegant way to solve this? Can we creatively think about what is *within* your control when it comes to you and others?

There might be at least two ways to approach this:

- First, what is in your control is to be there for others. That, you can do. There are most likely people around you and in your life that you genuinely care about. To what extent do they sense that?

- Second, you can become more aware of all the people who might already be there for you. To what extent do you sense their care?

Let us start by taking a closer look at the first approach: how to be that person for others.

The Wedding Speech, Part Two

What does "being that person for others" look like in practice? There are different ways of showing other people that you care about them. One skill that you can further develop to convey your care is empathy.

When we use the term "empathy," different people might have different associations with it. Therefore, let's first explore a practical definition of what empathy is and isn't through a thought experiment. To do this, we'll return to our wedding speech scenario from Chapter Two for an exercise.

EXERCISE 1
Where Is the Speech?

Now, imagine that you and your cousin have finalized the surprise wedding speech for your niece's wedding. In the months and weeks leading up to the wedding, you have

---

spent your rare spare hours writing, laughing, brainstorming, and rehearsing together. It's so great now that even your uncle is enthusiastic about it!

As the wedding draws closer, you get ready to get on the train. The wedding is far from home. You are excited and look forward to it. It's the first time that you've had a formal role at a wedding. You can't wait to see the bride and groom laugh at your jokes.

During dinner, on the night of the wedding party, your cousin seems to be missing. As the time for the speech draws closer, you get more and more nervous. Finally, five minutes before the time for the speech, he shows up and slowly walks up to you. When he reaches you, he pauses for a moment and then says: "Hey...I think we have a problem. You know the speech I was supposed to print for us to read from? I think I left it at home...in my other bag at home."

Instructions for This Exercise
Write down all the things you could say in that moment. You can write down what you personally would say or can imagine that someone else would say.

Now that you've written down everything that came to your mind, let's look at a simple structure by which you can analyze your responses.

Every communication between people contains at least two layers of information.

The first layer is easy to notice: it is the literal, verbal message. These are the actual spoken words, in this case: "Hey...I think we have a problem. You know the speech I was supposed to print for us to read from? I think I left it at home...in my other bag at home."

Then, there is also a second layer. The extra message, if you will. This is known as the emotional message, which conveys information about the emotional state of the communicator.

The way you deal with these messages can fall into one of the following five categories.[6]

Category One: Dismissing

One way of dealing with messages is to—for whatever reasons—dismiss the emotional message and perhaps also the verbal message. There are many situations where this can be a helpful approach. For example, think of moments of danger, urgent tasks, or crises when being decisive is all that counts. It is no coincidence that you'll see a lot of "dismissive" communication happening in hospital emergency rooms or military environments.

Here are some examples of Category One responses to the wedding speech exercise:

- "It's okay. No one knew that we were going to do this anyway."
- "What?! You idiot. I had emphasized three times to bring a backup. How could you be so neglectful?"
- "Oh wow. I saw this happen once in a movie. Do you know which one I'm talking about? The one with that comedian...what's his name?"
- "Don't you get how it will make me look if we can't give the speech?"

What do the above responses have in common? They are dismissive of the emotional (and, to an extent, even the verbal) message that your cousin is conveying. The messages are like balls that your cousin throws toward you, but you dodge them.

Category Two: Problem-Solving

Another way is to take the literal, verbal message, process it, and come up with a host of correct or incorrect, timely or untimely solutions for the issue at hand. It might not be a surprise that many problem-solving answers arise often and automatically: in school and at work, we are trained to become skilled problem solvers. As such, when we hear about someone's challenge or predicament, it can feel natural to ask: "How can we solve this?" or "What are our options?" or "How can I help?"

Here are some examples of Category Two responses to the wedding speech exercise:

- "Let's just improvise without the text."
- "Is there a printer in the area?"
- "Let's recreate it as best we can tonight and move the speech to tomorrow."
- "Shall we just forget about it and enjoy our evening then?"

Category Three: Acknowledging

A very different way of responding is to acknowledge the existence of the emotional message of the other person, even though its content might not be clear to you. By doing this, you open a door to their emotional world. It's like an invitation: the other person can decide to share a glimpse of that world or not—it's up to them.

Here are some examples of Category Three responses to the wedding speech exercise:

- "Oh gosh, how are you doing?"
- "How are you feeling right now?"
- "The speech isn't the most important thing to me; how are *you*?"

Category Four: Naming

Another way of responding is to not only acknowledge that there is an emotional message, but also attempt to name what that specific emotion might be.

You could be right, you could be wrong, but you try. The strength of this approach can be that it makes the other person feel psychologically visible, as opposed to only physically visible. When the other party cannot yet articulate their emotion, it can be a huge relief that you do. Even if the feeling you name does not reflect the other person's experience, you make it more likely for them to begin to articulate their feelings, and thereby, you also open up a space for intimacy to exist between you—if that is what they need from you.

Here are some examples of Category Four responses to the wedding speech exercise:

- "Oh, you must be sad..."
- "I can imagine you're upset."
- "Aren't you relieved that we don't need to give the speech anymore?"

Category Five: Contextualizing

A final way in which you could respond is to not only acknowledge and name the emotional message, but also put it into the context of the other person's life. This will be our practical definition of empathy in this chapter.

Here are some examples of Category Five responses to the wedding speech exercise:

- "I can imagine you're feeling sad because you worked so tirelessly on this on your weekends."
- "I can imagine you feel relieved, given how much you were dreading this...you often mentioned how you never liked public speaking."
- "You must feel angry, especially since you had asked me to print a backup version as well, rather than putting it all on you, as usual."

As you might notice, by adding context, you acknowledge this particular person, with his or her history, wishes, hopes, values, and dreams. You show them that you see how this moment fits into all of that.

Can you recall either giving or receiving a Category Five answer? What kind of effect did it have on you or on the other person?

It goes without saying that Category Five is not always per definition the best response. There is a time and place for each category. The main question is: are you responding out of choice or out of habit?

I Know *Exactly* How You Feel, and Other Pitfalls

What do you think the greatest mistake is that people make when attempting to offer empathy with the best intention? Imagine someone is in a crisis of sorts:

Scenario #1

Friend: "I feel a bit depressed..."

You: "I know exactly how you feel. I've been through the exact same thing. I'm going to tell you in detail what that was like, and also how I solved it."

Scenario #2

Friend: "I just got fired..."

You: "Hey, I know exactly what it's like. I've been there. I understand, totally, I lost my job once, too. But it's going to be just fine; look where I am now!"

How might these scenarios unfold? Your conversation partner might respond with something along the lines of: "Well...ummm...listen, you have no clue about how I'm feeling right now. When you lost your job, you didn't have my kids or my mortgage, so what you're saying really doesn't make any sense. Our situations are nothing alike." As a response, you might say something along the lines of: "Whoa, why are you reacting this way? You don't need to be so defensive! I was just trying to help!" And so on...

This happens when you imagine yourself to be empathizing, while in reality you're practicing well-meant, but misplaced, "relating." There are definitely moments where relating is appropriate. For example, relating is appropriate when you want to emphasize something you have in common with a stranger, or share tested solutions to a problem. Relating, however, is certainly not the same as empathizing.

The sad thing is that this situation could have brought two people closer together, but it didn't. It actually drew them further apart. An opportunity to strengthen their relationship was, instead, stranded in an off-topic debate about whose heartbreak, job loss, or defeat was worse.

As a simple rule of thumb:

Who is empathy always about? The other person.
Who is it never about? You!

And that's great news, because it means that you don't need to have had the exact same experience in order to have the right or the ability to empathize with another human being.

Going Full Circle

Let's go full circle. We defined a relationship as having someone in this world who cares about you. While this is outside of our control, it *is* within our control to be that person for others. Not in the cases where you genuinely don't care, but in all those situations where you really do care about someone and would like them to know.

The intent of this section is to create more awareness of the choices that you always have available to you, in each and every interaction in your daily life. When you want to show others that you care, you can do many things, such as solving their problem, relating to their situation, or empathizing with them.

Of course, doing the above may increase the chances of others also caring about you. However, as the ancient Stoics would say, that could be considered a "preferred indifferent": very welcome if it happens, but fundamentally not in your control and, therefore, not of concern.

As you practice this, of course, nothing stands in your way to do this for yourself as well. How often are you your own best friend? At the end of the day, after facing difficulties, how often do you ask yourself how you're feeling? Profoundly sad, sincerely relieved, overwhelmingly anxious, overcome with joy? How does that feeling fit in the context of everything else that is happening in your life? And can you offer yourself any creative solutions to deal with your difficulties?

Who Is Already There for You?

In the first part of this chapter, we discussed how it is within your control to be *that* person for others and yourself. What is also within your control is to—at least—be aware of who is already there for you. The good news is that you are most likely not starting from scratch. Chances are that there is already someone who cares for you—in the spirit of Athena. There might even be more people than you are aware of.

So, who is already there for you? And how easy or difficult do you make it for yourself to experience that? Let's try another exercise.

EXERCISE 2

Turning on the Lights

Take a few minutes to think about all the people in the world who could possibly care about you—either in your daily life or in the background of your life. These people could have a large impact on your life, or enrich it through small acts of kindness or support.

List these people's names and also, if you want, the ways that they are "there for you."

What was it like to do this exercise? How did it feel? Did anything or anyone unexpected come up?

At the outset of this chapter, we started with a strict definition of relationships: "someone in the world who cares about you." Now, let's stretch that definition a bit. Anyone who makes your life a bit easier, more joyful, and worthwhile may now also join the list.

These people could be family members, friends, acquaintances, classmates, neighbors, or colleagues. They could be human beings or pets. They could be alive or no longer here. They could be real-life people or fictional characters from books, movies, or poems. They could be people you encounter in person or people you've never met.

EXERCISE 3
Who Else Is Already There for You?

Who else would join the list if you stretched and played with the definition?

Feel free to pause for a moment. How did doing the exercise feel this time? Did anything surprising come up?

Who *Also* Could Be There for You?

Let's take a moment to think about how bonds between people form. Some people in your life may have been there from the day you were born or for as long as you can remember. All the other people have been strangers at one point in your life and somehow have now become part of it. How did this happen?

Most likely, the specific context in which you met each other was conducive to forming bonds: a context that repeatedly brought you back together, in settings where you could get to know each other better over time. Schools are good examples of such environments.

What does your current context look like? How does this "water" support the creation of new bonds or the deepening of existing ones? How comfortable are you with leaving this all up to chance?

EXERCISE 4

Deepening and Broadening

Take a few minutes to think about each of the following questions. This is an invitation to be as imaginative and creative as possible.

- Whom do you want to create a deeper relationship with? How could you achieve this?

- Who else would you like to add to your life? What could be a first step for this?

Chapter Four—Essence

Feeling cared for matters. While it is not within our control whether others care about us, it is within our control to be that person for others and ourselves.

Know what to do. When you want to show others that you care, you can do many things, such as solving their problems, relating to their situations, or empathizing with them.

Notice, deepen, and broaden. How easy or difficult do you make it for yourself to sense your current support group and to build it over time?

"Good thoughts, good words, good deeds."

—Zoroaster

Why & How

After being away from home for ten years fighting in the Trojan War, Odysseus and his men set sail to return. Despite Athena's help, their journey was still riddled with uncertainties. They had to outsmart dangerous mythical creatures, navigate difficult seas, overcome many strokes of bad fortune, and wrestle with the hands of fate. This journey home cost them another ten years of their lives.[1]

How did Odysseus sustain and endure that long journey with its countless hardships? One answer is that he had a very clear "why": to reach Ithaca and finally embrace his wife and his son once again.

In the spirit of Nietzsche: "He or she who has a why can bear (almost) any how."[2] Think back to the role models you chose in Chapter One. One reason they have been able to pull through, maybe even in the most challenging of VUCA times, is because they had a strong "why." Meaning, however, is not restricted to times of challenge and hardship. The good times in life also become richer when they have a sense of meaning to them. It can add color to our daily lives in beautiful ways.

As humans, we have been reflecting on the meaning of life, the stars, and the universe for as long as we can remember. Why are we here? Why are *you* here? These are profound questions that one can ponder on for an entire lifetime.

In this chapter, however, we will not try to answer the grand questions of life. Instead, we'll approach meaning with a radical focus on what we can control. The goal is to turn the ability to experience meaning into a practical muscle and to strengthen that muscle. How can you experience more meaning in seemingly ordinary moments of your day-to-day life? How can you create more meaning in your own life and in the lives of the people with whom you live and work?[3]

On Bricks, Pillars, and Schools

A person walked by a construction site and saw people at work. She walked up to one of the people and asked, "Excuse me, could you tell me what it is you're doing here?" He answered, "That's simple. I'm laying bricks." She walked up to another person who seemed to be doing the same and asked him the same question. He looked up and said, "That's simple. I'm building a pillar." When she asked a third person the same question, he said, "Well, I'm building a school. A place for kids to come and learn."[4]

For the lawyers among us, are any of these three people not telling the "truth"? Of course, this is a rhetorical question, and each person is sharing his view of reality. Nevertheless, one can imagine how the first person getting up to go to work might feel different than the third.

"Meaning" in this chapter is therefore not about the actual, externally observable reality but rather the inner, subjective experience of that reality.

The Most Meaningless Activity That Has Ever Occurred in Human History

To start practicing the ability to increase and decrease meaning in whatever you do, let's start with an exercise.

We will look at one single activity from three different angles:

- "Laying bricks," i.e., not contributing to anything
- "Building pillars," i.e., slightly contributing to something
- "Building schools," i.e., fully contributing to something of importance to you

Now, imagine a judge who, after delivering a verdict at the end of a big case that took months, has to sit for hours to write up her judgment for the official record. Let's discuss three different ways in which the judge can experience this activity.

0: Laying Bricks

What would she have to think to experience this task as "the most meaningless activity that has ever occurred in human history"?

- "Nobody is probably going to read it anyway."
- "I could do so many other things with my time."
- "I'm typing words at my desk."
- "Did I invest all those years to end up doing this?"
- "So many others could be doing this right now instead of me."

1: Building Pillars

Taking a different approach, how can we help this judge turn this activity into a (slightly more) meaningful experience?

- "Who knows, I might learn something new from this."
- "Doing this shows some dedication to my organization."
- "In case they are ever needed, I'll be relieved that we have these documents."
- "At least I'm practicing my writing and typing skills."
- "I'm helping out a busy colleague here."

∞: Building Schools

Now, how can we go overboard? How could we turn the judge's task into "the most meaningful experience that has ever occurred in human history"?

- "This can prevent a massive, unnecessary lawsuit that would have cost taxpayers money."
- "With this activity, I'm strengthening the trust in our constitution, which is the foundation of our society."
- "The template I am creating for the documentation of this case could serve as an example for my colleagues, saving them time and effort in the future."

- "A complete documentation of the case teaches me a lot about the case—I'm becoming a better judge for future, possibly more complex cases."
- "It is only by doing all aspects of my job correctly that I could be promoted to the highest court of our country."

Of course, this is just a thought experiment. But hopefully the point comes across: the same physical activity can be experienced completely differently depending on the level of meaning you attribute to it.

The above does not mean that, for any given activity, you should always go overboard and imagine it to be the most meaningful activity that has ever occurred in human history. It is mainly to show that decreasing and increasing meaning is something that is within your control.

When you want to increase meaning, you have the choice to turn on the lights and see what you're contributing to in all its richness: from creating something of significance to preventing something undesirable. Your task is not to try to see meaning in those places where barely any exists; it is to be sure you do not miss out on the meaning that may be present, because how would today be different for you if you could be able to experience more meaning in it?

EXERCISE 1

Full Meaning Workout

Now, it's your turn. Think of a recent activity you had to do that you didn't particularly enjoy.

How could you describe this as "the most meaningless activity that ever occurred in human history"? The equivalent of "laying bricks" (0)?

-
-
-
-
-

How can you make it slightly more meaningful (1)?

-
-

-

-

-

And how could you go overboard and describe it as "the most meaningful activity that has ever occurred in human history" (∞)?

-

-

-

-

-

Now, take a few moments to reflect:

- How did it feel to move through the three levels?

- What can you learn from this?

When Less Can Be More

One way that ancient Stoics were able to deal with potentially upsetting events was not by *increasing* but actually *decreasing* meaning: describing events as literally as possible.[5] When a special vase that has been in the family for generations accidentally falls and breaks, one way to experience this is as the destruction of the efforts of generations passing along a symbol of love, strength, and devotion. Another way to experience it is as a vase that fell and broke.

The Virtues of Yoda, Gandalf & Mr. Spock

When turning things into "the most meaningful activity," there is one often-overlooked realm that one can always contribute to: virtues. A virtue is a character trait that is considered positive.[6] In the past, many philosophies and schools of thought considered exercising virtues to be the main goal of human life.[7]

Let's return to our judge, who is still immersed in her paperwork. Our judge might realize that, independent of the external consequences of her work, she is also exercising virtues. Which could these be? Perhaps patience. For what are the only instances when one can practice patience? When one really, really doesn't want to, of course. Just as the only time to practice courage is in the presence of real fear. You can see challenging situations like these as occasions to practice virtues and thereby build your own character.

Every day, you make decisions under volatile, uncertain, complex, and ambiguous conditions. Independent of the outcome, under these conditions you are practicing the virtue of wisdom by thinking through the best course ahead. In doing so, you have joined the famous club of Yoda from *Star Wars*, Gandalf from *The Lord of the Rings*, and Mr. Spock from *Star Trek*.

Which virtues would you want to further develop? And what are the best situations to practice them in? To help you along, here are some common virtues that you could start with:

- Wisdom
- Courage
- Kindness
- Humility
- Diligence

- Honesty
- Patience
- Generosity
- Tolerance
- Compassion

Feel free to add any other virtues that come to mind.

-
-
-

-
-
-

EXERCISE 2

Practicing Virtues

Think about some of the activities that you have planned for the coming days. Are there any activities that you won't enjoy? What virtues could you develop through these activities?

-

-

-

-

-

"Let Me Explain It to You One More Time"

Everything that has been discussed so far can very well be applied to helping others experience meaning as well. However, there is an important point to consider before doing so. With all good intent, it is easy to overlook a simple truth:

> *That which is meaningful for you is not*
> *automatically meaningful for other people.*

Let's go back to our wedding speech example from Chapter Two, this time focusing on the content of the speech. Different guests may find the wedding meaningful for different reasons. Now imagine everyone were told that they should agree on only one good reason to be there (e.g., supporting the couple in love). How realistic would that be? And how necessary?

How often has someone else assumed that what he or she finds important must also be important to you? How did that make you feel? Looking back, how often might you have assumed the same about others?

So, how can we approach this question then? How can we distinguish between different sources of meaning and create space for them to coexist?

There are plenty, perhaps infinite, sources of meaning. There are also many ways to categorize them. For the sake of creating a shared language, here is one system of categorization.[8]

Categories of Meaning

	Examples
Personal	• Learning something new • Developing a virtue • Growing professionally
Relational	• Providing for the well-being of friends and family • Feeling a sense of belonging to a community, team, or organization
Organizational	• Strengthening an organization's performance • Creating an institution that lasts
Societal	• Restoring the environment • Exercising civic duties • Preventing harm to the economy • Building flourishing communities
Metaphysical	• Understanding fundamental life questions

Once you've read through these different categories of meaning, imagine that you've been given one hundred "meaning stars." Try to distribute them among these five categories based on what you find meaningful: not because you find them theoretically important, but because they truly excite you.

How was this? Did the answers come intuitively or did they require much thinking? Does anything about your distribution surprise you? Is it balanced or do you seem to have preferences?

Just as you might have preferences, so do others. Therefore, next time you want to motivate an entire group of people, your children, a classroom, your colleagues, or anyone else, you can be extra considerate about which categories of meaning you address. If you're not (in all your speeches, emails, questions, conversations, and celebrations), others might not tell you that your story doesn't resonate with them. They might just nod, because let's be honest—it's awkward to interrupt someone and say, "I really don't care about what you just talked about, your reasons, and the elaborate details you described." As you can see, this not only is a missed opportunity to infuse an activity with meaning but also can create an unnecessary distance between you and others.

Again, this is not about pretending that there is meaning when and where there might be none. Sometimes you just have a pile of bricks, and you need people to help you to lay them out. People will appreciate you being clear about that. However, with some practice, you might be able to provide the right amount of meaning at the right time for the right person, even with categories that don't directly resonate with you.

This doesn't mean you can't share what's meaningful to you with other people—on the contrary, this can actually be inspiring. Just be mindful of not universalizing your form of meaning and imposing it on all other human beings around you. Let's practice this in the following exercise.

EXERCISE 3

Tapping into All Sources

Think of a certain endeavor, task, or the start of a project that requires the help of other people to make it work. How could you present that story in such a way that it touches upon different categories of meaning?

Challenge yourself to see how far you can broaden each category of meaning toward infinity, while keeping it realistic.

0	1	∞
"Laying Bricks"	*"Building Pillars"*	*"Building Schools"*

- Personal

- Relational

- Organizational

- Societal

- Metaphysical

Discovering the "*Why*" That Can Help Bear (Almost) Any "*How*"

So far, you've learned how to navigate the spectrum between the utterly meaningless and the incredibly meaningful. You've also learned about different categories of what people can find important. This last exercise is meant to help you even further discover what's meaningful to you, based on your life so far.[9]

EXERCISE 4

Your Life

For each phase of your life, think of one, two, or three things that were important to you at that time. Allow this to be a free flow of memories, regardless of whether they are positive or negative, big or small.

Life Phase:

Important Thing #1:

Important Thing #2:

Important Thing #3:

Life Phase:

Important Thing #1:

Important Thing #2:

Important Thing #3:

Life Phase:

Important Thing #1:

Important Thing #2:

Important Thing #3:

Life Phase:

Important Thing #1:

Important Thing #2:

Important Thing #3:

Life Phase:

Important Thing #1:

Important Thing #2:

Important Thing #3:

How did this make you feel? Did you recognize any recurring themes or patterns? What could be the "why(s)" that have helped, and will continue to help, you bear any "how"?

It can be strengthening to know that many things you do certainly contribute to something larger than yourself. Perhaps, for some of those things, you will never see the end result. It might take more than one generation before the fruit of your work becomes visible. However, when it comes to meaning, every step can be seen as worthwhile in and of itself.

Chapter Five—Essence

Experience meaning. Not only by undertaking new or meaningful activities, but also by thinking differently about what you're already doing.

Acknowledge differences. It's completely possible to work on the same thing for entirely different reasons.

Apply now (or later). What is reading this book contributing to for you?

> *"The mystery of human existence lies not in just staying alive, but in finding something to live for."*
> —Fyodor Dostoyevsky

Start & Finish

~~~~~

Odysseus embraces his wife and son after twenty long years...

Heracles completes his twelve works...

Alexander finally understands what Diogenes means...

The construction workers finish building the school...

The two little fish understand what water is...

You have reached this far into this book...

While the previous chapter was about the journey, this one is about the destination.[1] It is about the senses of closure, completion, and achievement, however big or small. This feeling can be sought after for its own sake. Think, for instance, of someone who:

- Writes down a task on a "to-do list" after the task was already finished, just for the sake of being able to cross off the "to dos."
- Tries to win a game over and over again and finally does.
- Learns a new skill (e.g., playing an instrument, a sport, cooking a certain meal), just to be able to do it.

Is there anything that you do, purely for the "kick" that a sense of accomplishment brings? In the same way that food and water are physical necessities, a feeling of accomplishment can be considered a psychological necessity.[2]

Let's look at this in the VUCA context. How often do your surroundings provide you with a sense of accomplishment? Contrary to decades and certainly centuries ago, daily work for many is becoming increasingly abstract, intangible, and focused on the long term. Therefore, for many of us, moments of accomplishment do not naturally present themselves in our daily lives. Unless you are perhaps a surgeon or a shoemaker, it can take months or even years to see the final results of the work that you do every day. This can make it more difficult to pull through in challenging times.

EXERCISE 1

The Bar

Looking back on the past two months of your life, think of as many of your accomplishments as you can, and write them down. These can be things that are visible to others, or only to you. These can be things you accomplished by doing or, for instance, by "effortful not doing" (e.g., quitting something harmful).[3]

-

-

-

-

-

Some people, when doing this exercise, have just a few accomplishments on their list. Others have many. Does this mean that the latter group is much more productive than the first? The answer is obviously "no, not necessarily." But it does highlight that we all define accomplishments differently. And that's okay, because you are the only person who knows and can decide on whether you've truly accomplished something or not.

That's why you won't get a checklist for when something is an accomplishment or not. You can, however, become more aware of where you put the bar and why. Whether you want it or not, you do have a bar. How easy or how difficult are you making it for yourself and others to experience a regular sense of accomplishment?

What are the benefits of having a (very) high bar for what you consider an accomplishment?

- It can be an extra motivator to go beyond ordinary expectations.
- When you do achieve your goal, it might be more memorable.
- It could inspire others to do great things.

What is the cost of having a (very) high bar?

- You may risk never achieving your goals.
- It might prevent you from even starting a daunting task.
- You will rarely, if ever, feel like you have accomplished anything.

What are the benefits of having a (very) low bar for what you consider an accomplishment?

- You frequently experience the kick of accomplishment in your life.
- You enjoy continual boosts of motivation.

- It might be easier to start new tasks.

What is the cost of having a (very) low bar?

- It could dilute the quality of the kicks you get.
- You might feel less motivated due to a lack of significant challenge.
- It could distract you from accomplishing major tasks in life, leaving much of your potential untapped.

By reflecting on these questions, you can assess how you currently define accomplishment. Are there any adjustments you would like to make for yourself? In your view, does an accomplishment have to require willpower, or not at all? Is there anything that you would like to add (or remove) from your initial list? You could also ask people who are close to you what they consider your accomplishments to be.

Counting Colors

You might be sitting on a bench in the park reading this. You might be sitting on the bus or on a chair in your living room. Regardless of where you are, it's time to have a look around.

Count Everything That Is Red

You have exactly fifteen seconds to count the number of things in your surroundings that are the color red. Write the number below.

Now, write down the number of things that you saw that were *green*...without looking around again. :)

This exercise was obviously a bit of a trick to become aware of the effects of your focus. How many green things did you notice when you were counting the red ones?

The green and the red were both there, both at the same time. However, you mostly see that which you focus on. This analogy can be transferred to your daily life. What happens at the end of the week, if you ask yourself the following: What went wrong this week? What didn't I finish? What is still behind schedule?

These are perfectly legitimate questions, the equivalent of asking, "What was red around me?" But if you do not deliberately decide where to focus, you might end up only remembering the red. Or, you might end up believing that red was the most prevalent color in your surroundings. So how about in addition to—not instead of—asking yourself "What was red?" you also ask yourself "What was green?" In other words, at the end of the week, could you also ask yourself the following: What went well? What did I manage to finish on time? What went better than expected? This way, you can allow yourself to feel that kick, that sense of accomplishment, with each step that you take.

Magical Celebrations

Accomplishments can be dismissed, recognized, or, to make the most out of them, celebrated. In the words of the ancient Greek historian Polybius, "Those who know how to win are much more numerous than those who know how to make proper use of their victories."[4] Celebrations don't need to cost anything, nor do they need to be huge or preplanned. Spontaneous ones can even be the most memorable and fun.

Do you have any experience with celebrating accomplishments? What are some different ways you have enjoyed doing that? What would the people around you consider a nice way to celebrate their accomplishments? Could you help them in doing so?

EXERCISE 3
Celebration Ideas

What are some of your favorite ways to celebrate accomplishments? Below are some ideas just to get started—take some time to add your own.

- Get something delicious to eat.
- Play music that you love.
- Take a moment to do your favorite things (from Chapter Two).

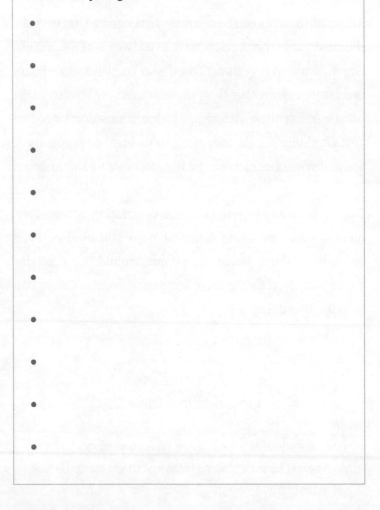

- Blow up some balloons and invite whoever helped you achieve your goal.

-

-

-

-

-

-

-

-

-

-

Congratulations! You have just finished the six main chapters of this book!

How will you be celebrating this?

Chapter Six—Essence

Successfully achieve things. In the context of a VUCA world, it is helpful to make the fruits of your work more visible to yourself.

Adjust the bar. You are the only person who can define what an accomplishment is for you.

Celebrate when you want to—starting now.

> *"Great acts are made up of small deeds."*
>
> —Lao Tzu

Love & Farewell

"Learning how to think...really means learning how to exercise some control over how and what you think. It means being conscious and aware enough to choose what you pay attention to and to choose how you construct meaning from experience. Because if you cannot or will not exercise this kind of choice in adult life, you will be totally hosed."

—David Foster Wallace

We started this book together with this quote, and we will also end with it, coming full circle. Everyone who has contributed to this book hopes that, in the process, you do feel like you have more choice, in any given moment, in any situation.

This book is not about what you *should* do, but what you *could* do. In the end, you can decide based on your own will, creativity, life experience, and unique strengths what you want to focus on. Whether it's the things that are in control or out of control, it's up to you. Whether or not it's increasing awareness of your environment and the people in it, it's up to you. Whether you want to focus more on your favorite things, being there for others, building your virtues, or celebrating how far you've come, it's all up to you.

The value of a vessel lies in its ability to take you across the river. Once you are on the other side, you continue with your life.[1] Hopefully this book has helped you along your journey so that you can get closer to where you want to be.

ACKNOWLEDGMENTS

Gratitude & Wonder

*"The highest to which man can attain is wonder; and
if the prime phenomenon makes him wonder, let him
be content; nothing higher can it give him, and nothing
further should he seek from behind it; here is the limit."*
—Johann Wolfgang von Goethe

Thank you to all those who ever wondered about life and
shared their thoughts with others. Like shining stars, these
thoughts can guide us in this changing world.

Thank you to Monireh Sadrzadeh, who, through her beautiful dreams, selfless efforts, and highest standards, made
everything possible in the first place.

Thank you to Leila Kian, who ever since our childhood has been a brilliant and creative companion in playing with the most colorful ideas: discovering, connecting, writing, naming, and rearranging them for fun and practical use.

Thank you to Clemens Fahrbach, who joined the Young Leaders Forum from the start, helped build a vibrant community, and went to great lengths to help with the creation of this book.

Thank you to Paulette van Ommen, my angel of inspiration, who, with her love, humor, and wisdom helped with each step of the way, especially during the most challenging times.

Thank you to all who kindly supported by opening doors: Claudio Feser, Sven Smit, Mary Meaney, Dominic Barton, Nick van Dam, Rob Theunissen, Dieuwert Inia, Peter de Wit, Wopke Hoekstra, Rik Kirkland, Pierre Gurdjian, Chris Gagnon, Paul Rutten, Jean Timsit, Gene Kuo, Corinne Pit, Rens ter Weijde, Fabian Billing, Marlies Zwaan, Scott Keller, Nikola Jurisic, Emmelie Erkelens, the great team at Scribe Media, Nicolai Nielsen, Miranda Berkhof, Cornelius Baur, Jakob Rüden, Anna Granskog, Martin Lösch, Jasper van Halder, Joanna Barsh, Matthias Breunig, Robert Carsouw, Allen Webb, Tori Fahey, Johanna Hirscher, Laurie Jansen, and Liz Ericson.

Thank you to all the friends and family who helped make things work, rain or shine: Noush Kian, Martijn Busstra, Annemiek Krans, Lennard Busstra, Manou Korst, Floris Busstra, Kim van der Feltz, Robin van Merkestein, Basia Kostrzewa, Kate VanAkin, Bryony Winn, Teun Hermsen, Tyson Gaylord, Sebastien Valkenberg, Mark Scheid, Sepand Samzadeh, Thibaut Pugin, Adeleh Hashemi, Glen Kruse, Juliette Audet, Simon Alfano, Anne Blackman, Hervé Huisman, Danelle Scholtz, Merja Kolehmainen, Josh Rothenberg, Marianne Moukhtara, Emilie Valentova, Muzi Yu, Emily Yueh, Parvin Samzadeh, Eman Bataineh, Audrey Stikkers, Jeroen Huisman, Marieke Ebbing, Faridun Dotiwala, Corentin Delépaut, Liza Rubinstein Malamud, Mohcine Ouass, Kevin Kumler, Joey Chin, Leonoor Schouten Netten, Tiffany Wendler, Maria Jos, Lisette Steins, Jan Tijs Nijssen, Christian Behrends, Corinna Gerleve, Jaap Vriesendorp, Jochen Hartmann, Julie Fry, Benedikt Krings, Alexander Bülow, Pekka Tölli, Meeke de Jong, Grace Ho, Mike Vierow, Hanna Kaustia, Kristina Thim, Martin Kramer, Adeline de Wazier, Ellen Bracquiné, Jean-Elie Aron, Alexandra McMurray, and Carol Weese.

About the Author

Kayvan Kian is an entrepreneur, teacher, and management consultant at McKinsey & Company in Amsterdam. He is the founder of the Young Leaders Forum and has given guest lectures at Harvard Business School, HEC, Sciences Po, and other schools. Ever since childhood he has been interested in understanding how some people are able to thrive through challenging times in life, and he hopes that by sharing these hard-fought lessons with each other, we can make this world a better place. He holds an MBA from INSEAD and a degree in both Economics and Law from the Erasmus University Rotterdam.

Personal Skill Matrix

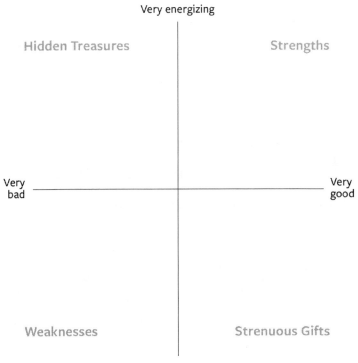

Very energizing

Hidden Treasures · Strengths

Very bad · Very good

Weaknesses · Strenuous Gifts

Very draining

Other Things within My Control

Other Things within My Control

Other Things within My Control

Other Things within My Control

Thoughts, Ideas & More...

Thoughts, Ideas & More...

Thoughts, Ideas & More...

Thoughts, Ideas & More...

SOURCES

H$_2$ & O

Introduction

1 M. Seligman, *Flourish: A New Understanding of Happiness and Well-being* (London: Nicholas Brealey Publishing, 2011).

2 The Young Leaders Forum is a multiday workshop developed by the author, designed to help young leaders lead, grow, and thrive in a volatile, uncertain, complex, and ambiguous world.

Chapter One: Awareness & Choice

1 E. Hamilton, *Mythology: Timeless Tales of Gods and Heroes* (New York: Grand Central Publishing, 2011).

2 D. F. Wallace, *This Is Water: Some Thoughts, Delivered on a Significant Occasion, about Living a Compassionate Life* (New York: Little Brown Book Group, 2009).

3 VUCA is a term first coined by the US military to describe the volatile, uncertain, complex, and ambiguous nature of our contemporary world.

4   B. J. Kreisman, "Insights into Employee Motivation, Commitment, and Retention," *Business Training Experts: Leadership Journal* (2002): 1–24.

5   J. Rodin, "Aging and Health: Effects of the Sense of Control," *Science* 233 (1986): 1271–1276.

6   P. E. Spector, C. L. Cooper, J. I. Sanchez, M. O'Driscoll, K. Sparks, P. Bernin, A. Büssing, et al., "Locus of Control and Well-Being at Work: How Generalizable Are Western Findings?" *Academy of Management Journal* 45, no. 2 (2002): 453–466.

7   Inspired by N. N. Taleb, *Antifragile: Things That Gain from Disorder* (London: Penguin Books Ltd., 2013).

8   Insight based on, and term coined during, conversation between L. Kian and K. Kian in Spring 2014.

9   Epictetus, *Of Human Freedom*, trans. Robert Dobbin (London: Penguin Books Ltd, 2010).

Chapter Two: Positive & Negative

1   Diogenes, *Sayings and Anecdotes, with Other Popular Moralists*, trans. R. Hard (Oxford, Oxford University Press, 2012).

2   Seligman, *Flourish*.

3   W. G. Parrott, *The Positive Side of Negative Emotions* (New York: Guilford Press, 2014).

4   M. M. Tugade, B. L. Fredrickson, and L. F. Barrett, "Psychological Resilience and Positive Emotional Granularity: Examining the Benefits of Positive Emotions on Coping and Health," *Journal of Personality* 72, no. 6 (2004): 1161–1190.

5   B. L. Fredrickson, "The Role of Positive Emotions in Positive Psychology," *American Psychologist* 56, no. 3 (2001): 218–226.

6   Used by permission of Hal Leonard Europe Limited, "My Favorite Things" (from *The Sound Of Music*). Words by Oscar Hammerstein II, Music by Richard Rodgers. © Copyright 1959 (Renewed) Richard Rodgers and Oscar Hammerstein II. Williamson Music, a Division of Rodgers & Hammerstein: a Concord Music Company, owner of publication and allied rights throughout the world. Print Rights administered by Hal Leonard LLC. All Rights Reserved. International Copyright Secured.

7   B. L. Fredrickson, "The Broaden-and-Build Theory of Positive Emotions," *Philosophical Transactions of the Royal Society B: Biological Sciences* 359, no. 1449 (2004): 1367–1378.

8   Insight based on and term coined during conversation between L. Kian and K. Kian in Summer 2017.

9   M. Seligman, *Learned Optimism: How to Change Your Mind and Your Life* (New York: Vintage Books, 2006).

10 The concept and terminology of learned optimism in this book is adapted and based on feedback from the Young Leaders Forum 2012–2019.

11 J. Gottman and N. Silver, *The Seven Principles for Making Marriage Work: A Practical Guide from the Country's Foremost Relationship Expert* (New York: Three Rivers Press, 1999).

12 Term inspired by title of the movie *Collateral Beauty* (directed by David Frankel and written by Allan Loeb, 2016).

13 A. M. Wood, J. J. Froh, and A. W. A. Geraghty, "Gratitude and Well-Being: A Review and Theoretical Integration," *Clinical Psychology Review* 30, no. 7 (2010): 890–905.

14 Term coined during conversation between L. Kian and K. Kian in Summer 2017.

Chapter Three: Strengths & Weaknesses

1 Epictetus, *Discourses, Fragments, Handbook*, trans. R. Hard (Oxford: Oxford University Press, 2014).

2 M. Csikszentmihaly, *Flow: The Psychology of Optimal Experience* (New York: Harper Perennial Modern Classics, 2008).

3 Seligman, *Flourish*.

4 M. Csikszentmihaly, *Flow: The Psychology of Optimal Experience* (New York: Harper Perennial Modern Classics, 2008).

5 J. Nakamura and M. Csikszentmihalyi, "Flow Theory and Research," in *Oxford Handbook of Positive Psychology*, ed. C. R. Snyder and S. J. Lopez (New York: Oxford University Press, 2002), 89–105.

6 This framework is adapted from CAPP—Strengths Profile, Gallup—StrengthsFinder, and Martin Seligman—VIA.

7 This framework is adapted from CAPP—Strengths Profile, Gallup—StrengthsFinder, and Martin Seligman—VIA.

8 J. S. Bolen, *Gods in Everyman: Archetypes That Shape Men's Lives* (New York: Harper & Row, 1989).

Chapter Four: You & Others

1 Homer, *The Iliad*, trans. R. Fagles (London: Penguin Classics, 1998).

2 Homer, *The Odyssey*, trans. R. Fagles (London: Penguin Classics, 1999).

3 Taleb, *Antifragile*.

4 Seligman, *Flourish*.

5 W. J. Chopik, "Associations among Relational Values, Support, Health and Well-Being across the Adult Lifespan," *Personal Relationships* 24 (2017): 408–422.

6   Adapted from J. Gottman, and J. DeClaire, *The Heart of Parenting: Raising an Emotionally Intelligent Child* (New York: Simon and Schuster, 1997); and R. Kegan, "The Colors of Emotions," *Counseling Master Class Handbook*, internal training material (New York: McKinsey & Company, 2013).

Chapter Five: Why & How

1   Homer, *The Odyssey*, trans. R. Fagles (London: Penguin Classics, 1999).

2   F. Nietzsche, *Twilight of the Idols* (North Charleston: CreateSpace Independent Publishing Platform, 2012).

3   Seligman, *Flourish*.

4   Adapted from the story of "John F. Kennedy and the Janitor" and the "Building Cathedrals" story by Annette Simons.

5   Epictetus, *Discourses*.

6   *Oxford Dictionary of English* (Oxford: Oxford University Press, 2010).

7   *The Stanford Encyclopedia of Philosophy*, s.v. Virtue Ethics (accessed 2016) https://plato.stanford.edu/entries/ethics-virtue.

8   Adapted from J. Barsh, *Centered Leadership: Leading with Purpose, Clarity, and Impact* (New York: Crown Business, 2014).

9   This exercise was originally introduced to the author by a colleague in Fall 2014 and is presented here in adapted form.

Chapter Six: Start & Finish

1   Seligman, *Flourish*.

2   Seligman, *Flourish*.

3   Term coined during conversation between L. Kian and K. Kian in Spring 2018.

4   Polybius, *The Histories*, trans. R. Waterfield (Oxford: Oxford University Press, 2010).

Conclusion: Love & Farewell

1   Inspired by the parable of the raft (Alagaddupama Sutta, verses 13–15), the Buddha.